Juicing Cleanse 3 Day Detox Diet

Easy 3 Day Diet Plan with Healthy Juices and Smoothie Recipes to Stop Sugar Cravings, Boost Energy and Feel Great.

Rebecca Hays

Copyright © 2013 Rebecca Hays All rights reserved.

No part of this book can be copied, or reproduced in writing without prior permission from the author.

ISBN-10: 1494411652
ISBN-13: 978-1494411657

Juicing Cleanse 3 Day Detox Diet

DISCLAIMER:
Any information in this book is for informational purposes and any use thereof is at your own discretion. The information presented without warranty expressed or implied, and is not intended to offer medical advice or treatment. Pregnant women, people with diabetes, eating disorder, on prescription medication, or with any chronic illness, or medical condition, should consult with their doctor before making any changes in diet or eating habits. Any health concerns should be addressed with your doctor or healthcare provider.

CONTENTS

1	Introduction	Pg 1
2	What is a Cleanse?	Pg 4
3	Benefits of a Cleanse	Pg 6
4	Why This Cleanse is Different	Pg 7
5	Juices vs. Smoothies	Pg 9
6	Macro-Nutrients vs. Micro-Nutrients	Pg 13
7	How to Juice	Pg 15
8	Create Your Cleanse Kit	Pg 18
9	Where to Buy	Pg 22
10	Why Eat Organic?	Pg 24
11	Stop Sugar Cravings	Pg 26
12	Tips for Success	Pg 29
13	Food Prep Tips	Pg 33
14	Ease In	Pg 43
15	3 Day Cleanse	Pg 45
16	FAQ	Pg 47
17	Ease Out	Pg 49
18	Juice Recipes	Pg 51
19	Smoothie Recipes	Pg 56
20	Vegetable Broth Recipe	Pg 60
21	Final Words	Pg 67

Rebecca Hays

In gratitude to my teachers.

1. INTRODUCTION

Welcome to the Juicing Cleanse 3 Day Detox Diet!

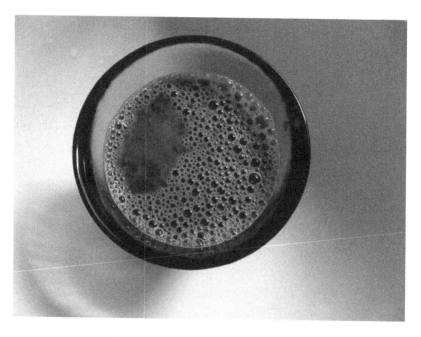

Congratulations on taking the first step towards a healthier you!

In this book you will find tips and advice plus a simple step-by-step guide on how to do a safe and effective 3 day juicing detox cleanse.

This powerful juicing cleanse includes more than simple juicing. See the section on Why This Detox Cleanse is Different. This gentle 3 day detox cleanse was designed by nutritionists for optimal health.

If you have juiced or cleansed before, or if you have never tried it, either way you will find this to be an enriching experience when you make the commitment today to stick with it, and do the cleanse.

What a powerful step to add years of healthy enjoyment to your life!

My first experience with a juicing cleanse happened after I had been sick for 3 days with the flu. I considered myself to be healthy and strong, but after being in bed for three days, barely able to drink water, I realized maybe my body was not quite up to speed. This is when I started juicing. I found it fairly easy to live on a liquid diet for a few days, considering I had not been able to hold down food the past few days!

But what happened to me was a HUGE surprise! By the third day of my juicing cleanse I not only felt better, but I had MORE energy than ever before! I could think more clearly. My body felt lighter. My mood improved. Even my vision seemed better (more on that later). I continued the cleanse for several more days, which was easy to do, because my old food cravings were melting away.

Of course, I did miss 'chewing' food, and after a week, I ate my first meal. A small salad. WOW! Even eating that small salad, I could FEEL a shift in energy. My energy dropped the moment I ate that salad. What an eye-opener!!

Eating a healthy salad, made my energy drop!!

How could this happen?!

The energy required to digest food is HUGE. Digestion steals energy away from everything else you want to do in life. This is one reason juicing is so powerful. Juice is much easier to digest than whole food. Just eating a small salad caused a tug on my energy, and slowed me down.

Benefits of Juicing

It was wonderful to notice, not only the increase in energy, but also how much FREE TIME I had when food was no longer a major focus of my life. It is amazing how much time we spend <u>thinking</u> about food. During the juicing cleanse, that all changes. I started getting projects done that had been put on hold. I even started to get rid of clutter!

And when the cleanse was over, I let go of some old habits, along with the clutter.

Everyone is in a different place along the path of life. Whatever brought you to this detox cleanse, you will find what you need, and get what is appropriate for you at this time.

Congratulations on making that commitment to yourself, to your health, and to your well-being.

Enjoy!

2. WHAT IS A CLEANSE?

Detox cleansing is a healthy way to amplify your bodies natural detoxification process. During a juicing cleanse you are drinking purifying juices, from fresh foods, which push everything else out of your system. It's a bit like spring cleaning (only you are spring-cleansing). Clearing out the pipes.

Our bodies automatically cleanse everyday. Detoxification is the body's natural process of eliminating and neutralizing toxins through the colon and liver. Your body even detoxes by elimination through the skin (the largest organ of the body).

The modern world puts so much stress on your body, you are exposed to a large number of toxins everyday, and the natural detoxification mechanisms in the body cannot keep up. Toxins get stored in the body in fat cells. When people lose weight those toxins are released.

The Juicing Cleanse is a specific 3 day diet plan that amplifies your natural ability to eliminate those toxins quickly and easily.

The Juicing Cleanse Detox Diet helps your body ramp up the natural detoxification process, at the same time, reducing the number of daily toxins entering the body. That's right! The food eaten by the average person contains what are considered 'toxins' such as added ingredients, GMOs (genetically modified foods), food coloring, dyes, preservatives, and other chemicals.

What does cleansing do?

Cleansing is a great way to kick-start healthy habits. It gives your body the chance to heal and repair digestive and detoxification pathways by providing nutrient dense foods in easy to absorb forms such as juice, smoothies and broths.

What should I expect?

Everyone's experience is different. Some people feel fabulous the very first day! Others feel a bit tired or have a slight headache. These are signs of your body detoxing. By the third day most people feel refreshed, re-energized, and are feeling better than ever before.

Will I lose weight?

Many people report mild to moderate weight loss. Keeping the weight off depends on the foods you eat after the cleanse.

Why this cleanse is fabulous!

After many years of trying various methods to cleanse and detox, this is one of my favorite cleansing detox methods. It is mild enough that the average person can do it, yet very effective in cleansing the body.

This 3 day cleanse will increase your body's natural ability to eliminate toxins, super-charge your immune system, and allow toxins that have been stored in your body over many years to be eliminated. By doing this cleanse you are bringing your body back into a state of natural health.

3. BENEFITS OF A CLEANSE

Benefits of The Juicing Cleanse 3 Day Detox Diet

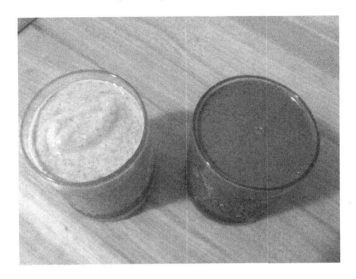

Benefits People Report after completing the Juicing Cleanse 3 Day Detox Diet

- ✓ Weight Loss
- ✓ More Energy
- ✓ Clear Thinking
- ✓ Better Focus
- ✓ Improved Digestion
- ✓ Loss of Cravings
- ✓ Feeling of Control over Mind and Body
- ✓ More Optimistic
- ✓ Better Mood
- ✓ Sense of Peace

4 WHY THIS DETOX CLEANSE IS DIFFERENT

There are many cleanses on the market today. Some include harsh supplements, herbs or medicine, and some require total fasting. I have experimented with a variety of cleanses, from intense to moderate to easy. This cleanse is geared to give you maximum benefit, without the extreme side effects that come about from more severe detoxification methods.

What I LOVE about this Juicing Cleanse 3 Day Detox Diet is the **unique combination of all natural ingredients.** If you are like me, you like food, and even though I love juicing, I also like to chew. The thought of living on juice for 3 days can seem a bit scary. Sure it's easy if you are coming off the flu, like I did the first time, but if you have been chomping down burgers and fries, or juicy steaks, the thought of a juice diet may seem overwhelming.

What I LOVE about this juicing cleanse is that it includes BOTH juicing and smoothies. There is also an optional De-Licious Broth, plus other steps to minimize any negative effects. Unlike a straight juice fast, the smoothies give somewhat of an 'illusion' of eating food. They have some bulk, and contain fiber to help fill you up. The broth contains enriching minerals to sustain you. The combination of juices, smoothies and broth give you everything you need each day to fulfill your caloric requirements.

It is normal to feel a little hunger on a cleanse, from time to time. But you will not be in starvation mode. If you have been an avid juicer for years, this may seem like a fairly easy cleanse. Great! Enjoy!

If you have never juiced before, it may seem like a bit of a challenge, yet still manageable. I like that this cleanse incorporates smoothies and broth, which help give the sensation of being satisfied.

In fact, I was surprised to find that most of the time, I was not hungry at all. I was THINKING about food but my physical needs were being met. (see the section on mental cravings) You will have everything you need as you detox your body with this juicing cleanse. And there are no harsh ingredients like some other cleanses. The most intense ingredient is the Detox Tea to assist with elimination, and this is optional (and may be swapped with Green Tea).

This juicing cleanse is designed to allow your body to naturally detox itself, by eliminating those toxins and impurities that enter the body everyday, and allow the body to heal itself. Combined with simple detoxing routines, you are using food to heal the body in a safe, easy and natural way.

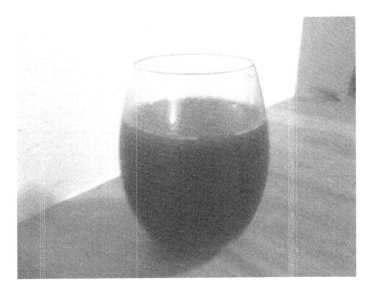

"Let food be thy medicine, and medicine be thy food"

…Hippocrates

5. JUICES VS. SMOOTHIES

When people think of juicing, they usually think of juice in a store. It comes in a bottle and has a nice deep color and very sweet flavor. It often has additional ingredients besides the fruit or vegetable, such as EXTRA sugar, flavoring, coloring, added dyes, and other chemicals.

This is NOT the type of juice you will drink in this cleanse. The juice you will enjoy will be made directly from PURE FRESH RAW FOODS, which give you the most nutrients, anti-oxidants, vitamins and minerals, packed into one small glass. If you have never juiced before, this is VERY important!

You're gonna LOVE it!!

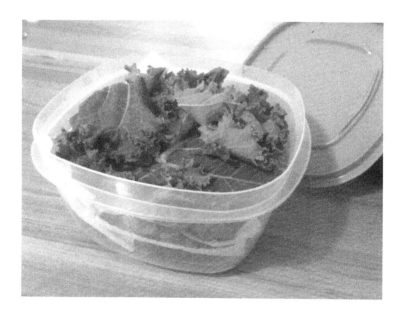

One of my clients came to me for coaching and decided to do a 'juice fast'. I later learned that her idea of a juice fast was going to a local health food store and buying bottles of pre-made juice. However, when she read the label she found all kinds of other ingredients besides food. Words she could not pronounce.

When you buy juice in a store, even if the only ingredient is the juice, that food has been PROCESSED in some way, which robs the food of nutrients. You literally cannot buy fresh juice in any store at any price, unless they are juicing those vegetables and fruits right in front of your eyes.

In fact, it is interesting to SEE how fresh juices do not look the same as those store bought juices that are supposed to be pure. They do not TASTE the same either! They taste BETTER! The first time I juiced grapes....the color was NOTHING like that deep dark purple in the store! But WOW! Super De-Lish!! Yum!

Why Not Just Eat The Food?

Because you won't.

You can take a full platter of veggies, and juice them into one single glass. You would have a hard time sitting down and chewing up all that food! Your mouth would get tired. You just won't do it. Juicing allows you to concentrate a large number of nutrients into a small glass of liquid energy that your body will soak up like a sponge!

What is a Juicer?

A juicer is not a blender. A juicer is a machine that extracts the liquid from fruits and vegetables, along with all the minerals, vitamins, antioxidants and enzymes, for a speedy delivery directly into your system. Juicing delivers a powerful nutritional punch, because it helps your body more easily absorb these phytonutrients.

Another Reason to Juice

The Juicer breaks down the cell walls of the food, releasing micro-nutrients and enzymes that your body needs. This fast release allows your body to absorb all those micro-nutrients instantly upon delivery. It also eliminates the first step in digestion, and skips that energy-drain on your body.

The juice you will be enjoying during this 3 day juicing cleanse comes from fresh food, both fruits and vegetables. If you continue juicing after the cleanse, you will be amazed, like me, that the fruit juices taste so incredibly delicious! You will never want to go back to store bought juice again.

What About Smoothies?

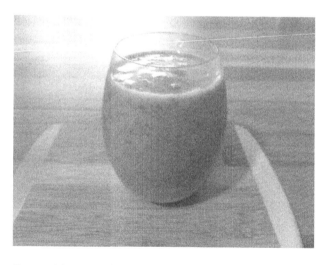

Smoothies are like juicing plus the pulp. Juicing will literally extract the nutrients and deliver them in a powerhouse liquid, while kicking out the fiber (called Pulp). Juicing gives you a pure liquid FOOD, without the pulp.

But it is also important to have fiber in your diet (and if you follow a strict juicing diet, you miss the fiber). By adding in smoothies in this 3 day detox, you are continuing to have fiber, which helps with elimination in the digestive system. Fiber also provides bulk which helps ward off hunger during the cleanse.

And with smoothies, once again, rather than eating whole, raw foods, which can be difficult to digest, just by blending the foods in the blender, you have begun to break down those cell walls, and release the enzymes and nutrients. Smoothies are more easily digested and absorbed into the body than whole foods.

Some opinions vary on juicing fruits because juicing gives you instant absorption, and with fruits, that also means natural sugars.

Please note that the majority of fruit in this cleanse comes in smoothies (a better way to consume fruits in general, rather than juicing). The fruits included in the juices are <u>very minimal</u>, and balanced with vegetables for the best result.

6. MACRO-NUTRIENTS VS MICRO-NUTRIENTS

If you are not convinced yet of the many benefits of juicing, I recommend you watch the movie <u>Fat, Sick and Nearly Dead</u> available on Amazon. The movie does a wonderful job of explaining macro-nutrients vs. micro-nutrients, in a fun and compelling way.

This book will not go into great detail but here's a quick overview.

Macro-Nutrients are foods like hamburgers, pasta, pizza, fast food, or ANY processed food that comes in a box, container, or plastic. Basically, anything that is not fresh, REAL food that grows in the ground has been processed. **Macro-nutrients are hard to digest** and cause a HUGE energy drain on your body. They take away energy from healing, they rob your vital energy to get tasks done, they make you feel tired. **Macro-nutrients are basically, energy thieves.**

Micro-Nutrients are foods like Fresh Juice from a juicer. They require very little digestive energy and are **easily absorbed by the body** very quickly. They send a burst of energy flowing through you. Micro-nutrients deliver important enzymes, vitamins, anti-oxidants and nutrients to every cell in the body.

Micro-Nutrients are like little healers for the body.

Some people experience an immediate effect when drinking juice, such as clearer vision. I had this experience one day driving down the highway, drinking my freshly juiced greens. Suddenly the signs on the highway became very sharp and clear, right before my eyes! As I noticed this and picked up my juice to take another sip, I thought, "Wow, this stuff really works!"

Cooked Foods

When you cook food, the heat robs some of the nutrients in the food. That means that fresh foods have the most vital nutrients, but fresh foods can be hard to digest. Your body needs enzymes to break down whole foods, which is why people take enzyme supplements. By juicing, you are breaking down the cell walls of the food, releasing enzymes and nutrients for immediate absorption.

Juicing does the digestion work for you!

Liquid Diet = Liquid Gold

And that means, juicing is one of <u>THE best ways</u> to deliver high-quality, potent nutrients to the body. That is why even a short, 3 day detox diet of juicing will have a powerful effect. Plus, the nightly broth delivers a delicious, mineralizing balance to round out your cleanse, and help keep you satisfied through the 3 day adventure. And finally, the luscious smoothies deliver vital fiber, to keep things moving, and help keep you satisfied.

7. HOW TO JUICE

Juicing can seem a bit daunting, or even scary at first. But once you get started, you will find it is very simple.

You will need a juicing machine. This is not a blender. It is a Juicer, made to extract the liquid nutrients, and spit out the pulp.

You can see a short video online about How to Use a Juicer.

To watch video go here: www.30secondsofbliss.com/HowToJuice

There are various types of juicers such as:

- ✓ Masticating
- ✓ Single Auger
- ✓ Twin Auger
- ✓ Centrifugal
- ✓ Cold Press

Higher end models give a higher yield of juice, especially with leafy greens. The price will range from $50 on the low end, to a few hundred dollars, or even in the thousands for the highest quality. But any type of juicer will work for your cleanse.

The juicer you buy will have easy to follow instructions. The basic idea is simple. You will purchase and prepare the food ahead of time. It will be much like putting food in a blender, but the difference is, your juicer will extract the minerals and nutrients into a liquid, and deliver them into a glass, fresh and ready to drink! At the same time the juicer will remove the pulp, the thick, fiber part of the food, and spit it out into a container.

You only drink the juice. Pulp can be put into compost, frozen for adding to a casserole or soup, or given to a neighbor to make homemade dog food. Pulp makes the best fertilizer for plants or the garden.

You want to drink your juice right away, or as soon as possible, because the enzymes begin to degrade once the juice is extracted. However, your juice can be stored up to 24 hours (or longer, depending on the type of juicer). For this cleanse, please drink your juice as soon as possible, on the same day that you prepare it.

Prepare your juice fresh everyday!

Whenever possible, drink right away!

To store your juice, put it in a sealed glass container, filled to the brim to avoid oxidation.

Purchase sealed glass bottles, or re-use glass bottles from your favorite drink. Just be sure to wash bottles thoroughly, and sterilize by rinsing with a small amount of hydrogen peroxide, or running them through the dishwasher.

If you drink Kombucha the bottles make great juicing containers.

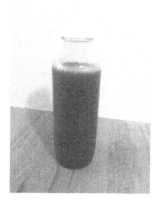

My Empty Kombucha Bottle Turned Juice Bottle!

Tips On Juicing:

- ✓ Let the juicer do the work. Do not PUSH the vegetables through.
- ✓ Juice 'slowly' to get more liquid from the food.
- ✓ After juicing, touch the pulp. If the pulp is wet, run the pulp through the juicer a second time, to get more juice.
- ✓ Alternate leafy foods with solids, to help push the foods through and get the most extract.
- ✓ Invest in a glass with measurements on the side that shows ounces. This will let you see how much juice you are getting.
- ✓ Check your juicing manual. Some juicers have two speeds for hard, or soft foods. Adjust the speed accordingly.
- ✓ Put a small plastic bag in the pulp container to catch the pulp. This lets you easily dispose of the pulp, without cleaning the container.
- ✓ Rinse the juicer under running water right away, and the food will rinse away easily.
- ✓ Be careful and do NOT touch the sharp blades with your finger when cleaning.

8. CREATE YOUR CLEANSE KIT

Your Complete Shopping Guide

Amounts are approximate, and depend on size of the produce, and yield you get from your juicer.

Note the evening broth is optional, or may be replaced with an additional green juice.

Juicing Shopping List:

12 carrots

1 large piece of fresh ginger root

1 jalapeno

3 oranges

6-7 Granny Smith green apples

6-7 cucumbers

3 lemons

2 pounds of fresh spinach

1-2 bunches fresh cilantro

2 stalks celery

2 bunches of fresh parsley

2-3 bunches of Kale

12 ounces coconut water (pure, no added ingredients)

Smoothie Shopping List:

3 fresh lemons

1 avocado

Hemp Powder

1 bunch fresh Kale

1 full head of organic celery

2 mangos fresh (or 2 cups frozen)

1 pineapple fresh (or 3 cups frozen)

1 small piece of fresh ginger root

1 small jar of pure almond butter

2 1/2 cups frozen organic cherries

2 1/2 cups frozen organic blueberries

1 small container cayenne pepper (or can buy 1 T in bulk)

Additional Items:

3 lemons for morning water

1 box detox tea, or green tea

Stevia, or honey to sweeten tea as desired
 (no sugar or artificial sweeteners)

1 multi-vitamin (recommend Source of Life Liquid)

1 bottle Probiotics supplement of your choice

Vegetable Broth (Optional, to have in evening, or may substitute this drink with an additional Green Juice):

2 T Olive Oil

25 whole Black Pepper Corns

1/4 tsp Cayenne Pepper

2 Cloves Fresh Garlic (peeled)

3 sprigs fresh thyme, or 1T cut up dried thyme

2 Organic Bay Leaf

2-3 T Sea Salt

7-8 Crimini Mushrooms

1 bunch of Organic Parsley

1 Leek (chopped)

2 lb Organic Carrots

1 Full Head of Organic Celery

Purified Water

If you do not have a water filter then stock up on plenty of purified water. Check your local store. Many grocers now have reverse osmosis filter water machines in their store. You can bring empty containers and fill them up for pennies.

DETOX BATH or Foot Bath

1 bag of Epsom Salts (Dr Teal's has aromatic essential oils added, such as lavender or Eucalyptus)

KITCHEN SUPPLIES

You may have some of these on hand, but this is a complete list that will get you through the cleanse.

- ✓ Juicer Machine
- ✓ Blender
- ✓ Lemon Juicer (hand held)
- ✓ Cutting Board Large
- ✓ Extra cutting boards, optional but helpful
- ✓ Sharp chopping knife.
- ✓ Small plastic bags for your juicer, to catch the pulp (optional)
- ✓ 16 ounce glass bottles with lids for storing your smoothies, juices and broth in the fridge.
- ✓ Large stock pot for making broth. If you don't have this, a deep dish pan with a lid would work too.
- ✓ Strainer
- ✓ Large Bowl
- ✓ Measuring spoons
- ✓ Sealed Containers for storing pre-cut vegetables in fridge (optional, or can use baggies)
- ✓ One rectangle shaped sealed container for storing celery (optional but useful)
- ✓ Freezer bags or small containers to put your pre-measured smoothie mixes into the freezer
- ✓ Teapot, or pan for heating water to make tea

9. TIPS ON WHERE TO BUY

Some people have the mistaken idea that juicing is expensive. I have been fascinated watching people check out at the grocery store and counted how many of the products they buy are real FOOD and how many are what I call **chemicals in a box**. So many people check out at the grocer without buying one single bit of real food.

Real food is food grown in the ground, then put into your shopping cart, without any processing in between.

But it can be interesting to notice how expensive those <u>macronutrient foods</u> cost. Have you ever filled up a grocery bag with meat and then checked the price tag?!! WOW!!

Load up a grocery bag with fresh vegetables and you may be surprised.

For the cleanse, whenever possible, buy organic. Even if the cost is more, for three days, it will be worth it. You are detoxing your body, so why would you introduce more unwanted chemicals into the body? And sometimes organic is about the same cost as non-organic.

Here are some tips on where to buy:

Farmers Markets are a great place to shop for fresh foods, which are typically organic, and you can often get a good deal there. There is even room for negotiation. Tell them you are starting a 3 day cleanse, and need to stock up, and if you enjoy the cleanse you will be back! Then gather up your produce and make them an offer.

Compare store locations. I was surprised to find our local chain grocery store, which has multiple locations around town, has different prices and selections at different stores. Some carry a larger supply of organic foods and some have better prices. Compare locations, shop around.

Juicing Cafes

You may be lucky and have a local store that sells fresh juice from a juicer (not pre-bottled, but made fresh to order). These are usually found in health food stores, grocers, cafes, or smoothie shops. If so, your juicing days have just become easier. You may not have to do your own juicing!

Juicers can be purchased online at Amazon, and several other places. They are now available in major stores, such as Target and Best Buy. You may even find a good deal on Craigslist, from someone who received a juicer for their birthday, and has it still in the box!

Or you may have a friend with an unused juicer stored in the closet. Ask around, you will be surprised.

10. WHY EAT ORGANIC?

A study by Newcastle University found **organic produce has 40 percent higher levels of nutrients, including Vit C, zinc and iron**, and a 2003 study in the Journal of Agricultural and Food Chemistry found **organically grown berries have 58 percent more polyphenols -** antioxidants that help prevent cardiovascular disease, **and 52 percent higher levels of Vit C** than non-organic.

Choosing organic produce increases nutrients, and, lowers your exposure to pesticides.

Since the purpose of the cleanse is to DE-TOX the body…adding more chemicals to the body is counter-intuitive.

However, depending upon where you live and your access to food, it may be difficult or even impossible to find organic foods.

If you have to buy non-organic foods, you will still benefit your body by doing the cleanse.

When Do I Really Need to Buy Organic?

The Environmental Working Group's Shoppers Guide to Pesticides identifies fruits and vegetables that have the highest and lowest pesticides.

The **Dirty Dozen** are the top 12 foods found to have highly toxic pesticides, and are the foods you would want to buy organic whenever possible.

If you would like to see the complete list of the Dirty Dozen, go to this website: www.30secondsofbliss.com/dirty-dozen/

For the cleanse we recommend you buy only ORGANIC for the foods found to contain highly toxic pesticides.

Buy these foods organic, to avoid toxic pesticides:

Apples

Celery

Spinach

Cucumbers

Kale

On the flip side, certain foods were found to have the lowest traces of pesticides, and may be safer to eat non-organic.

These foods are better choices for non-organic:

Pineapple

Avocado

Mangos

Mushrooms

Tips for non-organic foods:

Peel non-organic foods before juicing. For leafy foods, Kale, Spinach and others, buy organic when possible.

Wash produce thoroughly with running water and soak in vinegar water for a safe and thorough cleaning.

Remember, even though your favorite store may not carry organic, the very same store across town may have a nice selection. Check around. Look for farmers markets. Check the frozen food section for organic fruits. Buy your vegetables FRESH.

11. STOP SUGAR CRAVINGS

If you are like me, and LOVE chocolate, ice cream, or other sweet foods, then you realize how difficult it can be to STOP eating those foods that add pounds, a belly roll, and send a big knock to your health and immune system.

Sugar addiction has become a key word with my coaching clients that want to stop the sugar cravings. But how?!

Any food craving is a combination of both body and mind.

The craving can be physical; your body learns to want more of that food.

And also a mind-game; your mind is dreaming up Disney-Animated-Color Movies of sugary treats that appear larger than life!

Reducing and eliminating sugar from the diet is a process that evolves, and depending where you are on this path, it evolves like this:

1. Over-Eating Refined Sugars and Carbohydrates (white flours, white sugars, includes processed foods, buns, breads, cakes, sweets, fast foods)

2. Eating those same foods in moderation

3. Eating less refined sugars and more Natural Sugars (fruits, some vegetables)

4. Eating minimal amounts of sugars, mainly through fresh produce such as fruits, and some vegetables

5. Totally eliminating sugar from the diet

While total elimination of sugar is both rare, and difficult to do (requires constant maintenance) you can greatly reduce the amount of sugar. Remember that sugar is in almost every single box, package, processed food that you buy, and goes by over 20 names (hidden ingredient). Carbohydrates are also basically sugar in the body (white flours, breads, cakes, buns, pastas, all those type of foods).

Two ways to break a sugar addiction are:

1. Eat LESS of the bad stuff and,

2. Add in MORE of the good stuff.

With the 3 day juicing cleanse, you are doing both. You stop eating refined sugars for 3 days, and also start teaching your body to crave real, healthy micro-nutrients (which it does naturally anyway).

Realize that stopping any habit is a process. To break that sugar habit, do this:

- ✓ Repeat the 3 day juicing cleanse once a month.
- ✓ When you finish the 3 day cleanse, continue to enjoy a green juice every day.
- ✓ You might even enjoy a smoothie everyday too!
- ✓ One month later, do it again.
- ✓ Rinse and repeat.

You will find old habits gradually fall off, and better habits take their place, as you retrain your mind and body to crave natural healthy foods. Soon your body will crave the natural sugars in the smoothies (fruits) instead of refined sugars.

When this happens, you are shifting in the right direction.

After you have eliminated refined sugars from the diet, you can begin to reduce the total amount of natural sugars, and add in more vegetables instead. Juicing (and smoothies) are a good way to do this.

After my second time of doing the cleanse, my cravings for chocolate ice cream (my favorite!) had disappeared! When I imagined chocolate ice cream, I could only imagine a big box of chemicals (which it is) and the creamy cayenne smoothie seemed much more appealing!

Anytime in the future that the sugar habit returns, which can happen, simply return to the cleanse, and reboot once again.

12. TIPS FOR SUCCESS

MAKE IT EASY

Because as you know, when something is easy, you are more likely to do it.

This 3 day cleanse is as much a mental game, as it is physical. If you find yourself, like me, driving along salivating at every fast food joint that passes you by, even those you never liked before. Or walking through a park and suddenly the thought of creamy nachos pops into your mind, wondering where in the heck did that come from?!

Then you will quickly learn that these are temporary weak moments that I call <u>mind games.</u> This is your <u>mind</u> wanting food, not your body! During one of those weak moments, if you needed to start chopping a load of vegetables and clean them up and assemble a juicer, you may find yourself tempted to dive head first into a bag of cookies instead.

Preparation is Key.

<u>Have everything ready ahead of time.</u>

When you begin to feel hungry and the juice, or smoothie, or broth, is there just waiting for you and all you have to do is drink it…you WILL.

See Section on Food Prep Tips for a summary of how to prepare everything in advance.

Plan the Date

You could jump into the cleanse at a time when your best friend is throwing a huge BBQ party, or having a Pasta-Gorge Feast Dinner Party! But why torture yourself? Plan the date to happen when it is easy. Begin when you have a day off, or even two. With nothing to do.

If you do have a social (food) engagement, just take your juice with you (in a cooler). Brag about how cool you are, for being in control of your health.

Be Good to Yourself

This cleanse really is as much a mental game as it is physical. This is a good time to cleanse not only your body, but also your mind.

During the cleanse you will be surprised how much FREE time you have on your hands, when you are not constantly obsessing about food.

<u>Use that free time for a mental cleanse:</u>

As you prepare your food, think good thoughts

Tell yourself how proud you feel doing something good for your body

Go for walks outside

Take Epsom salt baths - add 1 cup Epsom salt to warm water

Take Epsom salt foot baths - add 6 tsps of Epsom salt in a footbath or dishpan with warm water and soak your feet, which removes toxins

Meditate

Sleep

Journal - write down your thoughts and feelings

Hunger

Realize that it is normal to have occasional feelings of slight hunger on a cleanse. But these are no worse than when you are watching an awesome movie, and realize you skipped lunch. In that moment, the hunger pain kicks in, but you stick with the movie, because it is worth it!

Remember:

Hunger is felt down in the stomach, in the gut. But...

Mental cravings are in the mind.

They are a thought, an idea, a concept.

They are not even real..they are <u>imaginary!</u>

They may be an image in the mind (ooh....creamy sauce!)

Or a taste or a smell (yum, ice cream..hot bread)

<u>Good news:</u> **A mental craving can be stopped, by turning your attention somewhere else. Because it is <u>just a thought.</u>**

Clear the clutter. Tackle that project. Go for a walk. Take a nap. Turn your attention away from food.

Anytime you feel hungry do this…

1. Drink a glass of water.

2. Drink more juice.

3. If you are very hungry, nibble on a small salad.

4. You can also nibble on celery sticks, or carrot sticks. Take small bites, chew slowly and fully. And STOP eating when the hunger stops.

5. You can also take a nap.

Make it a Spa-Moment…

Make Day One a Spa-Moment! Take the day off. Go for Walks. Sleep. Relax. Enjoy. And feel good about doing something special for yourself.

13. FOOD PREP TIPS

To Make the Cleanse Easier - Prepare In Advance

Clean, wash, dry, and chop all vegetables and fruits so they are ready to go into your juicer, or smoothie. You can prepare all veggies and store them the night before the cleanse begins. Freeze the fruit.

Prepare the broth before you begin and it will last all week. Optional, you can replace the evening broth with an extra green juice.

**Prepare smoothies the night before you drink them.
Prepare the juice each morning on the day you will drink it.**

Purchase airtight containers for keeping vegetables fresh.

I have one long rectangle shaped container for Celery...

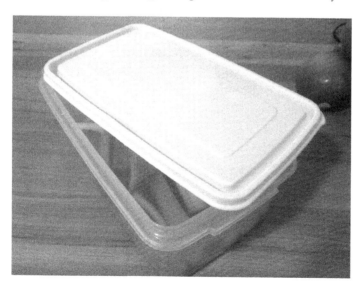

and a few large square containers for Spinach and Kale...

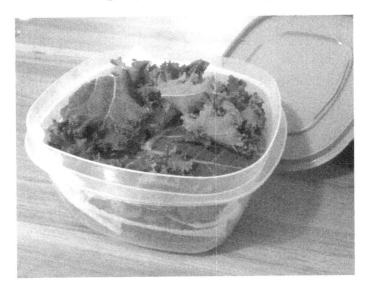

Celery

Wash the celery with a veggie brush and water. Cut in strips to fit into your juicer or blender, and store in the refrigerator in a sealed container filled with water. This will last through your cleanse, and be a quick and easy grab.

Kale

Wash the Kale under running water. Spread out on cutting boards to dry, or blot with paper towel. Once the Kale is dry, pull off the outer leaves (removing the spine) and store in the sealed containers.

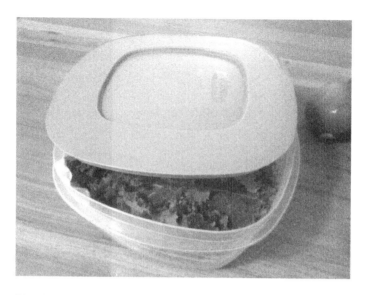

Fresh Kale, Cut n Ready to Go!

Make sure the Kale is dry and it will last the entire 3 days. Put paper towels between layers to absorb any additional moisture. For juicing, you can use the entire Kale, spine and all. For smoothies, remove the spine.

Cucumbers

If you purchase non-organic cucumbers then peel the outside. Organic is fine to juice the entire cucumber, just wash thoroughly.

Pineapple

You can buy pineapple already frozen and cut (be sure to get organic, no added ingredients) but fresh pineapple is both fun and de-lish!

If you have never cut into a fresh pineapple it can seem a bit daunting the first time, but it really is easy, once you get the hang of it.

There are gadgets that will core the pineapple for you, but a sharp knife will do the job. Choose a pineapple that is slightly brown or turning brown.

First cut off the top with all the green leaves, and then the bottom. Use a large cutting board, as juice will fly. Then slowly rotate the pineapple around, cutting off the outside brown edges. Slice off the pineapple fruit around the edges, leaving the thin core in the middle.

Cut the pineapple into 1 inch chunks, and spread out the chunks on a cutting board. Then put this in the freezer, so the chunks freeze into <u>individual</u> chunks, like ice cubes.

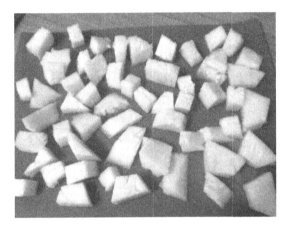

Pineapple Chunks, Ready to Freeze

If you freeze the chunks in one big container they will stick together and become one large block of ice. You will have quite a time trying to break them apart! After the chunks are frozen, you can move the frozen chunks into baggies or containers

Mango

You can purchase mango frozen (get organic, with no added ingredients) or prepare fresh.

Choose a Mango that is a little soft. Peel, cut and Freeze using same method as the pineapple.

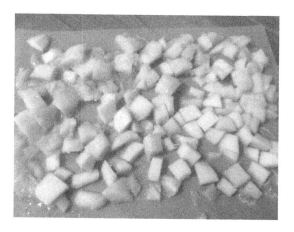

Mango Chunks, Ready to Freeze

Ginger

Cut ginger into one inch chunks. Cut off the outside peeling. Freeze. Frozen ginger breaks apart fairly easy, and you can freeze it in one container.

King Kale Smoothie Tip

Put frozen ingredients together in one container or freezer bag to make a pre-measured smoothie mix. That way you have one container with your smoothie mix, ready to go!

Just drop the mix in the blender. Voila! This let's you make a <u>really quick smoothie</u>. This one step will save time when you are in a rush, on a busy day.

King Kale Smoothie Pre-Mix

1/2 cup mango, 1 cup pineapple, and 1 ginger cube per bag or container.

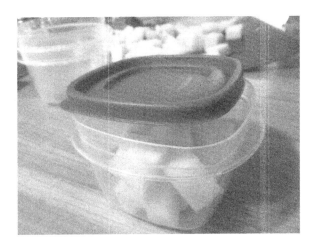

Pre-Measured Fruit Mix for Smoothie

Blueberry and Cherry

These can be purchased fresh, or frozen. If frozen, be sure they are pure organic, no added ingredients. Cherries are easier purchased frozen, without the pits.

Cayenne Berry Smoothie Tip

Similar to the the King Kale Smoothie, you can pre-measure and mix your cherry/blueberry fruit together in one baggie or container, ready to go in the freezer, for a faster smoothie mix the next day.

Cayenne Berry Smoothie Pre-Mix

3/4 cup blueberry and 3/4 cup cherry

Avocado

Before this cleanse my response to avocados was "I do not like them". But I was amazed at how good they taste in the King Kale smoothie, and they have a ton of beneficial properties for your body. When you buy an avocado find one that is a little soft. One avocado will get you through the cleanse. Slice it with a knife from top to bottom, and make another slice a quarter way around the avocado. Then just peel off that section, and dig out the soft food inside.

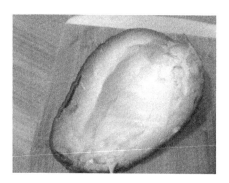

Water

Please use filtered, purified, or distilled water throughout the cleanse. Use this for drinking water, in your tea, in your smoothies, and if you add it to dilute your juice. If you do not have a purifier or filter, then stock up on bottled water at the local store. Purchase by the gallon and get a better deal.

Many stores now have machines that let you bring your water bottles and fill them up for a very small fee. These machines use reverse osmosis and provide very clean drinking water. You can save empty gallon jugs, take them to the store, and refill for pennies. Your body will thank you!

Coconut Water

There are many brands, and some have additives. Read the label. Look for pure coconut water with the lowest sugar content (coconut water has a natural sugar content) and make sure it does not have any other ingredients.

Spinach

Spinach can be cleaned and stored similar to Kale. Many stores now sell fresh organic spinach in pre-packaged plastic containers, ready to go. Transfer to a sealed food container to stay fresh longer.

Lemon

The juice of a lemon is best squeezed from a fresh, organic lemon. Stock up on these, as you will use one in each smoothie, and in your water each morning. You can purchase a very inexpensive hand juicer for lemons. This will come in handy.

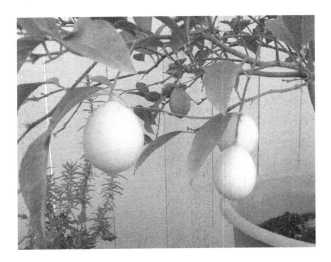

If you prefer, you can juice all of your lemons at once, and then measure out 2 T to equal one lemon. However, the juice from lemons is best FRESH, as the enzymes are active when fresh squeezed. If possible, juice your lemons fresh with each serving.

PREPARE Smoothies the Night Before

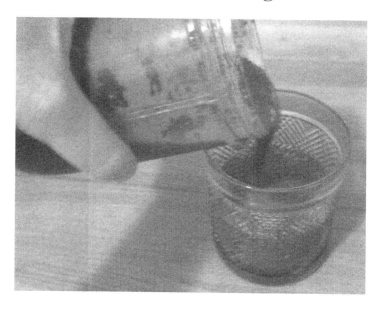

Prepare your 2 smoothies the NIGHT BEFORE. This was a life saver for me. In a moment of temptation, as images of fast food and fries are dancing in your head, if the smoothie is there in the fridge ready to go, you are more likely to drink it. If you have to pull out a bunch of food, chop, clean and prepare, then you could end up diving into a bag of potato chips instead! Store your smoothies in sealed glass containers in the fridge and they will be delicious the next day.

Glass Bottles

A simple tip is to re-use your favorite glass drinking containers. After drinking many Kombucha's the glass bottles were filling up my recycle bin. I realized they make PERFECT water bottles for on the go! But they also make the perfect juice or smoothie bottle. They are exactly 16 ounces (smoothie size).

You don't have to be a Kombucha drinker to use this trick. Glass bottles are best (because plastic leaches toxins). Begin saving any of your favorite glass containers that have re-usable lids. You can use coke bottles, tea, energy drinks. Sixteen ounces for smoothies, and ten ounces for juice. You could use Mason Jars, or any glass jar. You can also purchase glass containers with airtight lids. Have enough on hand to store all your smoothies, juices and broth.

Juice can be stored in glass containers for use the same day. Juice is best served within about 10 minutes of prep, as the enzymes are most active then. Over time, the enzymes react to air (oxidation) and lose potency. If possible, drink your juice right after juicing.

Juice - Drink - and THEN clean the juicer!

If you are super- busy and on the go, you can make all your juice each morning. Drink your first juice, and put the rest in bottles in the fridge. Fill the bottles to the brim, to avoid oxidation. Just be sure to drink juices the same day you prepare them. If you take them with you, keep them in a cooler.

The broth can be made before your cleanse even begins. It will stay good in the fridge for about a week, and up to a month in the freezer. You can make the broth during your Ease In period, and be ready to go. If you are super-busy, you can buy a container of all natural vegetable broth, but your homemade broth will have more nutrients than store bought.

14. EASE IN

What to do Before the Cleanse

Before jumping into a cleanse, head first, you want to get ready.

I made this mistake once long ago when I did a cleanse that was very intense. Thinking I could handle anything, rather than EASE in, I JUMPED in Head First, and then, BOUNCED right back out!

I felt so bad the first day, I quit.

My mistake was my belief that... "I can eat all the ice cream I want, chug down my last bit of caffeine late into the night and really ENJOY all this fattening food one last time, before starting my cleanse tomorrow!"

Big mistake!

Here is how you do it the right way rather than the way I did it back then.

Begin to make some of these changes in your diet a week, or at least 2 days, before the cleanse.

Start drinking more water.

Start eating more vegetables (if you eat zero, then any will be an improvement).

Cut back, or eliminate, sugar. If you eat half a gallon of ice cream a day, cut down to one cup. Then stop.

Cut back on caffeine. If you drink 6 cups of coffee a day, cut it to 3, then to 1.

Stop eating fast food, <u>completely.</u>

Cut back on processed foods (anything in a box) and start eating more salads and fresh foods.

This will allow your body to adjust to the changes you are about to make, with ease.

If you have never juiced before, begin to enjoy a daily juice a few days before the cleanse begins. Start by juicing pure granny smith apples. They are delicious, and will help you cut out other sugars.

For BEST RESULTS 1 week, or a minimum of 2-4 days before the cleanse reduce or completely avoid the following:

- ✓ Caffeine
- ✓ Alcohol
- ✓ White Foods: sugar, dairy, white flour, processed/packaged food
- ✓ Over the Counter Medication, unless prescribed by your physician

15. THREE DAY CLEANSE
Daily Schedule

(Recipes Listed at the end of this book)

Upon Rising (6-8am)

Drink warm glass of water with 1 fresh squeezed lemon, and

1 cup of Detox Tea, or Green Tea

Breakfast (7-9am)

Drink one Green Juice (10 oz)

Take one Probiotic supplement

Mid-Morning Snack (9-11am)

Drink Any Juice of your choice (10 oz)

1 cup Detox Tea (may replace with Green Tea)

Lunch (11am-1pm)

Drink One King Kale Smoothie (16 oz)

Take Multivitamin

Mid-Afternoon Snack (2-4pm)

Drink one Green Juice (10 oz)

1 cup Detox Tea

Dinner (5-7pm)

Drink One Cayenne Berry Smoothie (16 ounce)

Evening Snack (6-8pm)

Drink Vegetable Broth (10 oz), or

May substitute one Green Juice (10 oz)

Evening Detox Bath

Soak in warm bath with 1 cup Epsom Salt at least 10 min (may also add 1 cup apple cider vinegar)

Alternate Option:

Soak feet in tub of warm water with 3 tsps of Epsom Salt

Nurture yourself while cleansing!

- ✓ Take nightly baths, or soak feet in Epsom Salts to relieve sore muscles and enhance relaxation.
- ✓ Walk outside 30 minutes to increase circulation and oxygenation.
- ✓ Use this opportunity to connect to nature. Increased oxygen flow helps eliminate toxins.
- ✓ Get a massage to assist with lymph flow and total body relaxation.
- ✓ Meditate to become aware of your own body and the world around you.
- ✓ Keep a daily journal to write any thoughts or emotions that arise during the cleanse.

16. FAQ

What if I feel hungry?

It is normal to feel a bit hungry during a cleanse. The cleanse is designed to meet your basic caloric needs.

If you are using more energy than you are consuming, Eat!

Drink more water. Drink more juice.

Eat raw, fresh veggies such as carrots, celery, or green leafy vegetables to support your cleanse process.

Eat only enough until you are 'not hungry' and then stop.

What to do if you have headaches?

Drink more water

Take 500mg to 1000mg of Vitamin C

Drink another 6-8 oz of green juice

Take a nap

Can I exercise on the cleanse?

Yes. Mild to moderate exercise is fine. Listen to your body.

Walking and stretching are excellent to help your body eliminate toxins.

Strenuous exercise is not recommended.

What to do after the cleanse?

Use this cleanse as a kick-start to healthy habits, including diet, exercise, and positive thinking about yourself and your body.

Continue enjoying a daily juice for health.

Plan to reboot with a cleanse periodically to maintain optimal health.

See the Ease Out for instructions on the days following the cleanse.

17. EASE OUT

What to do After the Cleanse

Congratulations!! You made it through the 3 day cleanse! Your body thanks you! You are Fabulous!!

Breaking a cleanse correctly is just as important as the cleanse itself.

To maintain that healthy glow, you do not want to jump back into fast, fried foods, which also equal fast fat.

Here is a simple recipe for ending the cleanse.

Days 1 to 3:

Begin by eating fresh salads, lightly steamed vegetables, fresh fruits, nuts, or soups.

Have 3 light meals a day.

Continue to enjoy a green juice each day.

Add in other juices to enjoy.

Days 4 to 6:

Begin to add in whole grains as you wish, including brown rice, quinoa, beans or legumes.

Avoid white flours, white sugars.

Continue to enjoy a green juice each day.

Day 7 and Beyond:

You may add in dairy (optional), such as plain yogurt and eggs.

You may slowly reintroduce meat, poultry, tofu, or fish if you wish.

Continue juicing each day.

Plan on balancing your diet with at least 50% fresh, raw foods (juicing is an easy way to do this).

Tips for Easing Out

Chew slowly and thoroughly to digest food easily.

Stop eating before you are full.

Avoid overeating.

When adding back foods such as wheat, dairy, gluten, or sugar, notice any reactions the day you eat the food.

Notice any changes in energy, digestion, cravings or other symptoms with foods you add into your diet.

Eat foods that have natural detox properties from the Top 20 Natural Detox Foods.

For a FREE DOWNLOAD Listing the Top 20 Natural Detox Foods go to this website:

www.30secondsofbliss.com/top-20-detox-foods

18. JUICE RECIPES
For Your Cleanse

All of these juices are filled with cleansing, detoxing foods for optimal health.

GREEN JUICE #1: Love Cleanse

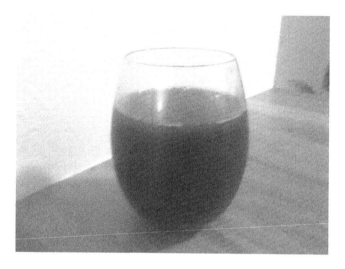

1/2 large cucumber (or 1 small)

2 celery stalks

4 cups Kale

2 cups parsley leaves

4 cups spinach

4 ounces water, or coconut water (optional, as desired for personal taste)

Yield: 10 ounces of juice.

TIP: For a higher yield from Leafy Greens, alternate with celery and cucumber. When you run the celery/cucumber after the kale/spinach/parsley it will help you to produce more juice from those greens.

Note:

Different juicers give different yields of juice. You may need to adjust the amount of produce depending upon your juicer. Adjust to taste.

GREEN JUICE #2: Margarita Detox

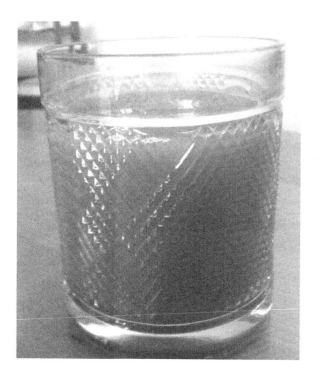

1 cucumber

1 granny smith apple

1 lemon

4 cups spinach

1-2 cups fresh cilantro

1 cube of ginger

Yield: 10 ounces of juice,

TIP:

For a higher yield alternate spinach/cilantro with cucumbers/apples. When you run the cucumber/apple after the spinach/cilantro it will help you to produce more juice from those greens.

Note:

Different juicers give different yields of juice. You may need to adjust the amount of produce depending upon your juicer. Adjust to taste.

BONUS JUICE #3: Serene Sunrise

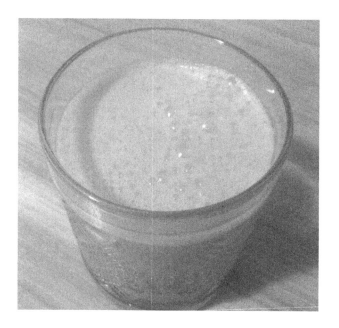

4 carrots

1 cube of ginger

1/4 to 1/2 jalapeno

1 orange

1 granny smith apple

Yields 10 ounces of juice for a single serving.

Enjoy <u>up to one of these per day,</u> as it has a higher sugar content, or you may choose to stick with all green juices for your cleanse.

19. SMOOTHIE RECIPES

Smoothie Recipes For Your Cleanse

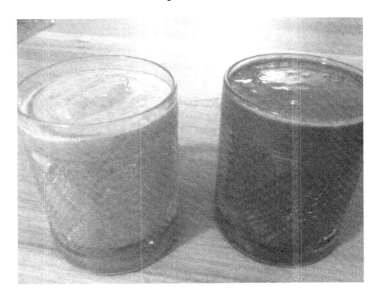

INSTRUCTIONS FOR MIXING ALL SMOOTHIES

In a blender:

1) First blend liquids (water, coconut water, lemon juice)

2) Second blend powders, spices, nut butters, or avocado

3) Third blend unfrozen foods (kale, celery, avocado)

4) Add frozen foods last, a few pieces at a time, and blend fully.

ENJOY

King Kale Smoothie

This smoothie is designed to have anti-inflammatory properties with healthy caloric content and balanced sugar intake.

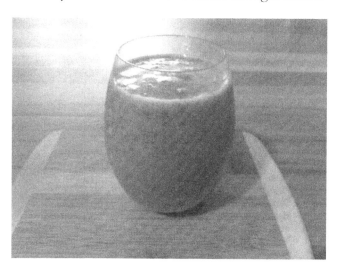

1/2 cup Filtered Water or Coconut Water (may increase or decrease as desired)

Juice of 1 Fresh Lemon

1/4 avocado

2 T. Hemp Powder

2 Kale Leaves (with the spine removed)

3 ribs of Celery

1/2 cup Frozen Mango pieces

1 cup Frozen Pineapple Pieces

1/2 inch frozen Ginger cube

Makes 16 ounces. Mix per instructions above and Enjoy!

Cayenne Berry Smoothie

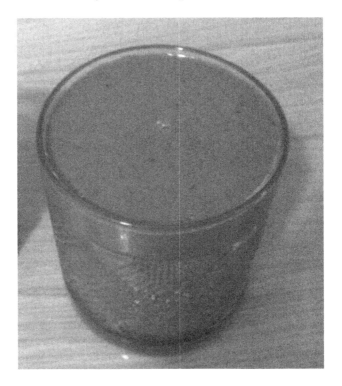

This smoothie will help satisfy that 'sweet tooth' during your cleanse and the ingredients provide many natural health benefits.

- ✓ Anti-Cold and Anti-Flu
- ✓ Anti-Fungal and Anti-Bacterial
- ✓ Digestive Aid
- ✓ Detox Support
- ✓ Joint-Pain Reliever
- ✓ Bone Health
- ✓ Supports Weight Loss
- ✓ Lowers Blood Sugar
- ✓ Promotes Heart Health
- ✓ Healthy Immune System
- ✓ Brain Food

Cayenne Berry Smoothie

Ingredients:

1/2 cup filtered water, or optional coconut water (slightly increase or decrease amount for desired consistency)

Juice of one fresh squeezed lemon

2 scoops of Hemp Powder

1 T. Almond Butter (get pure almond butter, no added ingredients)

3/4 cup cherries, frozen

3/4 cup blueberries, frozen

1/8 tsp cayenne pepper

Makes 16 ounces.   Mix per instructions above and Enjoy!

20. VEGETABLE BROTH RECIPE
For Your Juicing Cleanse

The savory broth recipe is designed to bring a rich, mineralizing balance to the cleanse experience. This vegetarian broth is nightshade free, gluten and dairy free, and avoids many of the food triggers for people with food sensitivities.

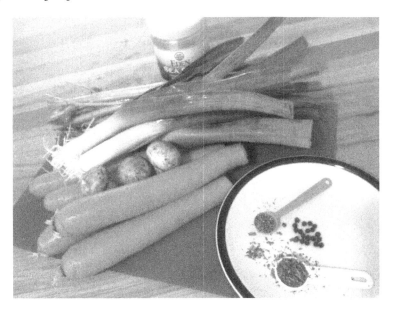

Note:

To receive the true benefits of your cleanse, enjoy making your own broth. Even if you have never cooked before, you will find it very easy to follow the recipe below. And with each serving you will feel good knowing you have done something special for yourself.

By making your own broth, you will fill the kitchen with a wonderful smell, and fill your body with an enriching superfood, and perhaps have an enjoyable experience too!

You can make the broth ahead of time (before you start the cleanse). It will keep for one week in the refrigerator. If you absolutely cannot make the broth, then purchase a pure vegetable broth without added ingredients. Either way you will benefit.

Base:

6 cups filtered water

2 T Olive Oil

Spices:

25 whole Black Pepper Corns

2 Cloves Fresh Garlic (peeled)

1/4 tsp Cayenne Pepper

3 sprigs fresh thyme, or 1T dried thyme

2 Organic Bay Leaf

1-3 T Sea Salt (to desired taste)

Veggies:

1 Leek (chopped)

2 lb Organic Carrots (chopped)

1 Full Head of Organic Celery (chopped)

7-8 Crimini Mushrooms

1 bunch of Organic Parsley

Heat a large stock pot with 2T of Olive Oil in the bottom, over medium heat.

Thoroughly clean, and then chop, all veggies. Add the veggies into the pot as you go. Chop the Leek, toss it in.

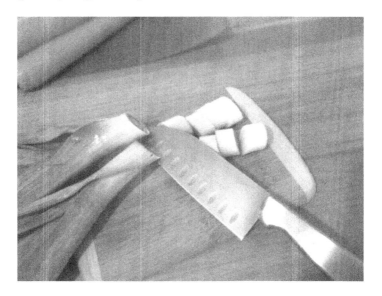

Chop the Carrots, toss them in. Chop the Celery toss it in. Chop the mushrooms and parsley toss them in. Stir occasionally as you are chopping.

Then add the spices.

TIP: To easily peel the garlic clove, do this:

Put a single clove under the knife, with the wide, flat side of the knife on top of the clove.

Bang on top of the knife with your hand, pressing down on the garlic

This loosens the garlic skin. Then cut of both ends of the garlic clove, and the skin easily comes right off!

Add 6 to 8 cups of filtered water. Your pre-made broth may look like this.

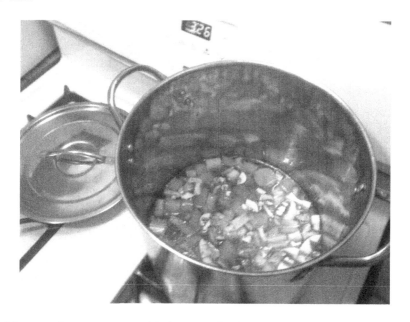

Turn up heat, cover and bring to a boil.

Upon boiling, turn down heat and simmer for one hour (stir occasionally)

Then uncover and simmer another 20-30 minutes to seal in the flavor.

After an hour the broth takes on a brown color and a rich flavor.

The simmered broth looks like this.

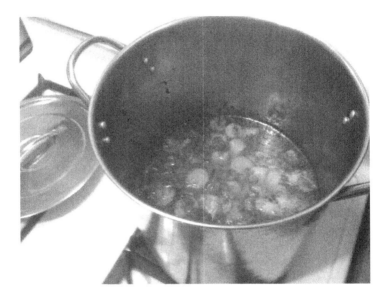

You may taste, and continue to simmer longer if desired. The longer you simmer, the stronger the flavor.

Strain broth through a strainer into a dish or pan. You may further strain the broth through cheesecloth if desired.

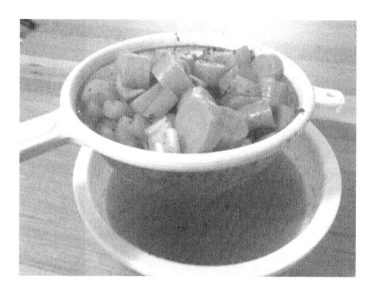

Pour broth into 3 glass containers, 10 ounces each, and store in the fridge. You are ready for your nightly broth!

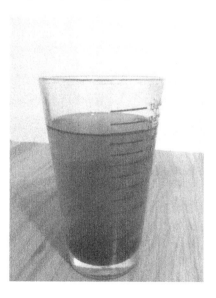

Super cool glass with ounces marked on the side!

The broth will keep for up to a week in the refrigerator.

BONUS Free Report
Top 20 Natural Detox Foods

After your cleanse, maintain your health by adding naturally detoxifying foods into your diet.

These detox foods enhance your bodies natural ability to cleanse each day.

For a FREE DOWNLOAD Listing the Top 20 Natural Detox Foods go to this website:

www.30secondsofbliss.com/top-20-detox-foods

21. FINAL WORDS

Congratulations on completing the Juicing Cleanse 3 Day Detox Diet!

The steps you have taken in the past few days have gone miles towards improving your overall health and well-being.

You may return to this cleanse, three or four times a year to maintain optimal health. Some people do the cleanse each month.

Remember to eat foods that help your body detox naturally everyday.

Get the FREE List of the Top 20 Detoxification Foods and start adding them into your diet.

To get the Free Download go to this website:

www.30secondsofbliss.com/top-20-detox-foods

If you have enjoyed this book, please return to where you purchased the book and write a positive review. Thank you.

To your health!

...Just The Beginning

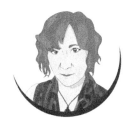

ABOUT THE AUTHOR

Rebecca Hays is an author, producer and artist with a broad range of interests. Certified in NLP, Hypnosis and Reiki, she has an ongoing interest in the mind-body connection and holistic healing. She runs a private coaching practice, along with classes and workshops, and produces media in various forms for personal development and spiritual growth. Her favorite challenge and personal growth experience is her yoga practice.

Rebecca began juicing long ago, after being knocked down with the flu. She was amazed at how quickly her body healed, and how absolutely fabulous she felt. She has been an avid fan of juicing ever since.

For more info visit the website: www.30secondsofbliss.com

Attribution

The following images were supplied by Creative Commons License:

Picture of Lemons: http://bit.ly/18zIWX3 by Elaine with Gray Cats

Picture of Green Juice Cup: http://bit.ly/180zM2f by William Ismael

Made in the USA
Coppell, TX
13 February 2022